# THE LIFE & TIMES OF

# Florence Nightingale

BY

Esther Selsdon

SHOOTING STAR PRESS

This edition printed for, Shooting Star Press Inc, 230 Fifth Avenue, Suite 1212, New York, NY 10001

Shooting Star Press books are available at special discount for bulk purchases for sales promotions, premiums, fund-raising or educational use. Special editions or book excerpts can also be created to specification. For details contact – Special Sales Director, Shooting Star Press Inc., 230 Fifth Avenue, Suite 1212, New York, NY 10001

This edition first published by Parragon Books
Produced by Magpie Books Ltd, 7 Kensington Church Court, London W8 4SP

Cover picture & illustrations courtesy of: The Florence Nightingale Museum Trust London; Mary Evans Picture Library.


ISBN 1 57335 048 6
A copy of the British Library Cataloguing in Publication Data is available from the British Library.

Typeset by Hewer Text Composition Services, Edinburgh
Printed in Singapore by Printlink International Co.

# EARLY YEARS

Fanny and William Nightingale gave birth to her first daughter, Parthenope, in Naples the year after they were married – 1818. Mrs Nightingale, who was a fine society lady and adored parties and nightlife, had heard that the city of Florence was, at that time, the most fun-loving in Europe and so she could not resist. She persuaded her altogether more serious husband to hire a villa there and it was on May 12 1820, in this house that Fanny gave birth to her second daughter and immediately decided to christen her after the gaiety-filled place of her birth.

Fanny herself was descended from a remarkable line of liberal-thinking people. Her grandfather, Samuel Smith, had given up his title to a large proportion of the city of Savannah, in the United States, in order to show his support for the American citizens during their War of Independence. Her father, William Smith, was, in his day, a leading political lobbyist and campaigner on such burning contemporary issues as the abolition of slavery and factory workers' pay. He tried to bring all ten of his children up to share both in these high moral aims and in his energetic love of life and, in fact, none of them died before the age of sixty-nine. Fanny, although the beauty of the family, remained for a long time uninterested in what she thought of as silly young men but, suddenly and quite out of the blue, at the ripe old age of 29, she fell madly in love with the Honourable James Sinclair, a young nobleman with no income who had no intention of marrying her. Fanny pleaded in vain that she would rather live for love with no money than live without him as a wealthy woman but he was not to be persuaded. Fanny was lovelorn and almost thirty. Along came William Edward Nightingale, a rather haphazardly youthful and intellectual friend of her brother's and almost twenty-four. He was besotted with the beautiful Fanny and, having come into a fortune at the age of twenty-one and seeing his opportunity lying ripe before him, he asked for his beloved's hand in marriage.

Even at that early stage she felt no real interest in W.E.N. but she was heartbroken about James and so, in desperation, she said 'yes'. At this early stage he tried hard to please his fiancée and his generally reserved and philosophical temperament underwent a temporary transformation – as Fanny was later to remark "Mr Nightingale is seldom in the melting mood". Fanny's family did not approve of the bizarrely thoughtful William but she believed that she could reform her husband and make him into a less high-brow and more approachably domestic man. Straight after the wedding she took him abroad for almost three years of travelling in Italy but, though William caught the bug and would have been happy to live a wandering tourist's life forever, Fanny, eventually, wanted to return home and, as was to be the way for much of their life together, her will prevailed.

W.E.N. was an amateur architect and he conceived the idea to design his young family a new home. It was called Lea Hurst and Fanny hated it. Although it had fifteen bedrooms, she considered the house isolated, cold and small. Fanny refused to live in her husband's dream home and forced him to buy another house, Embley Park, which was on the borders of the New Forest in Hampshire. From this spot Fanny could visit her sisters easily and would, therefore, not have to spend so much time alone with her husband and, by the time Florence was five, the Nightingales' life had developed into a fixed pattern in which they spent a few months of the Summer at Lea Hurst and the remainder of the year at Embley Park.

Twice a year they paid a quick visit to London, which is where Fanny would have lived constantly given the choice but at which her husband drew the line and it was, therefore, into this domestic regime that Florence grew up.

She was a strange child. Her mother considered her obstinate and morose. She was obsessed by the idea that, secretly, she was a monster and that this fact might, at any moment, be discovered. She worked herself up into paroxysms of terror if forced to welcome strangers to the house and she refused to dine in company. She wrote that, as early as the age of six, the affluent lifestyle into which she was born was hateful to her. As she grew older she ceased to be terrified and began to despise it and, although she hated meeting new people and never felt the slightest affection for her mother, she developed a series of embarrassingly intense passions for a variety of older women to whom she clung with temperamental vehemence – her governess Miss Christie and W.E.N.'s younger sister Mary were just two of these. When the women got married and moved away from Florence, which they all eventually did, she would make herself physically ill and refuse to come out of her bedroom for days.

She did, however, adore her charmingly intellectual and scatterbrained father although she was, herself, a meticulously tidy and methodical girl. When she and her sister were twelve and thirteen respectively, they made a pact to get up early every morning and to teach Bessie, their housemaid, to read and write. Parthe was keen on the idea but never actually managed to get up. Florence pursued the plan with methodical meticulousness. The sisters were close but incompatible. W.E.N. noticed all of this and decided that it would be impossible to find a governess suitable for both girls and that he must, therefore, take on this responsibility himself. He taught the girls Latin, German, French, Italian, history and philosophy and Florence loved every minute of it. Parthe hated the whole military regime. By the time Florence was sixteen she was W.E.N.'s constant companion in the library whilst Parthe had given up on formal education and learnt to arrange flowers in the drawing room with Fanny.

In the summer of 1834 the family's quiet, country life was shattered by the news that W.E.N. had been asked to stand for parliament in Andover. He had always said that he would never enter politics until the Reform Bill of 1832 became law but, once it did, he jumped in to the arena with grand ideas for change and unbridled enthusiasm. Since, however, he refused to bribe the constituents he was not only defeated but retired profoundly disillusioned. Fanny was mortified. She had thought that, at last, she might get the house in London for which she had longed her whole life but knew now that this would never happen by means of her failure of a husband. She gave up on him and transferred all of her plans and ambitions to her daughters who, being sixteen and seventeen, must soon "come out" in society. The Nightingales simply must add six more bedrooms to Embley in order to make it presentable and, in the meantime, the whole family would travel to Europe and educate the girls in the ways of the truly civilised world.

Florence, as a teenager, was lonely and intellectually isolated. Her mother and sister were mentally and emotionally miles away from her but her father was unapproachable. The younger Miss Nightingale hoarded paper obsessively and, angst-ridden, wrote long and intimate notes to herself. In February, 1837, when she was not yet seventeen, she became convinced that the answer to her anguish lay in some kind of spiritual salvation. "Today God spoke to me", she wrote, "and called me to His service." She was, apparently, convinced that she had heard real, external voices, and that they had summoned her to do some kind of unspecified but charitable good. The voices told her nothing definite but she became sure that she could only achieve peace of mind through following the call of God and, for the first time in her life, she felt confident and full of faith.

On September 8th, 1837, the Nightingales crossed from Southampton to Le Havre and began their voyage of cultural discovery in an enormous travelling carriage designed especially for the purpose by W.E.N. himself. Its interior was fully kitted out with special gadgets for comfortable eating and reading and the roof was fitted with seats for servants. Florence was in raptures – this was the most romantic thing that had ever happened to her. Each day, in her journal, she noted with meticulous precision exact hours of departure and arrival and precise mileages covered. The family travelled on as far as Nice and it was here that Florence

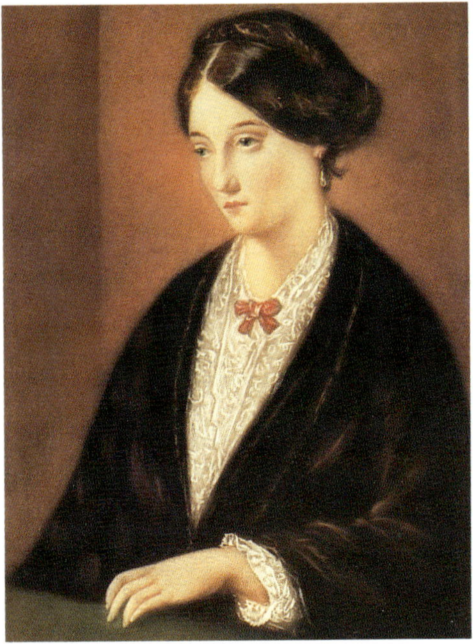

Florence Nightingale

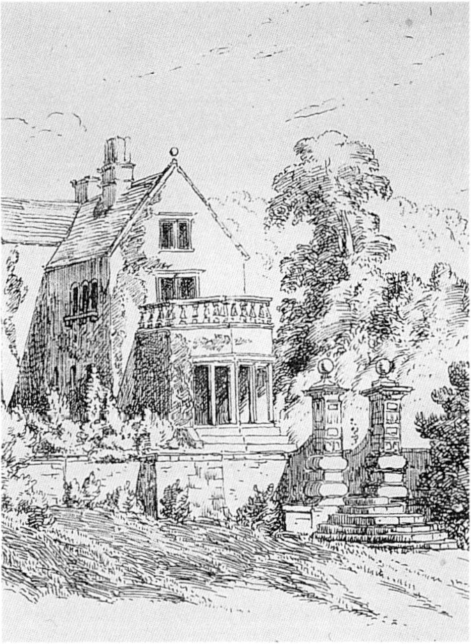

Lea Hurst

developed her passion for dancing. They moved on to Genoa, which, of all the places they visited Florence preferred, since, here, life was choc-a-block with balls and "she had so many partners that she became confused. An officer came up and challenged her in a rage because after refusing to dance with him, she sat out with someone else and there was an 'embrouillement'". This was all a far cry from Embley and Florence had never been so enraptured with life until, at last, in February, the Nightingales reached Florence – the intellectual and artistic capital of Italy. Florence was ecstatic. She went to the opera three times a week and she became a vocal advocate of Italian freedom, whose importance was impressed upon her a little while later in Geneva where the family met well-known figures from the Italian revolutionary movement – all now ruined and exiled for their progressive views and values. This was an enlightening experience for Florence since never before had she encountered people who were so aristrocratic and so cultivated and yet so painfully poor. She could not understand it.

Eventually the family moved on to Paris where they hired an apartment in the Place Vendome. It was, wrote, Fanny, "extremely splendid" and, via a letter of introduction from her sister Patty, she endeavoured to have her whole family introduced to one of the most celebrated women in Paris – Mary Clarke. Though unattractive, Mary Clarke had still contrived to become one of the most eligible women of her time. She knew everyone, including the famous philosopher Chateaubriand and his friend Madame

Récamier. It was a well recognised fact, however, that Mary Clarke did not like women, "Why don't they talk about interesting things? Why don't they use their brains?" she was frequently heard to say, and yet she immediately warmed to the entire Nightingale family and particularly to Florence. The pair met almost every day and Mary introduced the whole family to everyone she knew. Florence was wildly happy. She was passionately attracted to the woman the Nightingales had christened 'Clarkey' and she was intrigued to observe that, although Clarkey met her friend, Claude Fauriel, every day and that the pair were devoted to each other and that Fauriel treated Clarkey as an intellectual and emotional equal, still they were not married and yet this intimacy was accepted by society without question. This was an astonishing eye-opener for Florence and, with it, she came to believe that it was possible for a woman to be close friends with a man without provoking a scandal. It was a belief which stayed with her and was to regulate her conduct throughout her life. Florence was, all in all, very happy but she did realise that her life was trivial and, by April 1839, in any event, it was time to go home. At this stage it was two years since God had spoken to her and, just before she left Paris, she wrote in a note to herself that, to make herself worthy to be God's servant, the first temptation to be overcome was "the desire to shine in society".

In April 1839, however, Fanny and William Nightingale were totally unaware of their daughter's secret aspirations and congratulated themselves on the possession of a charming and gifted young daughter destined for a brilliant social success. Embley was still not fit for habitation at this stage and so the Nightingales decided to stay on in London for the whole 'season'. On May 24th, Florence and Parthe were presented at the Queen's Birthday Drawing Room. Florence wore a white dress she had bought in Paris and she looked radiant. The girls were caught up in a maelstrom of excitement and, once more, Florence's "call" vanished from her mind. She became seized with a passion for her cousin, Marianne Nicholson and wrote "I never loved but one person in my life, and that was her". But Marianne was unpredictable, volatile and needlessly cruel. She toyed with Florence's emotions right until the Nightingales went back to Embley and she enjoyed it. A short while later, back at home, Florence became furiously discontented with life, in general, and Marianne, in particular. Hampshire county society was inexpressibly dull; Marianne infuriatingly unaffectionate. Florence once again made herself unwell. She refused to come out of her bedroom where she spent her time studying mathematics, philosophy and Greek. She plagued herself at length and she blamed her volatile heart for her unworthiness before God.

By the winter of 1843 Henry Nicholson, the brother of Marianne, had become Florence's fervent admirer. He pressed her to accept his hand in marriage and Marianne railed at Florence for not not accepting him. Florence was heartbroken by what she saw as Marianne's deliberate cruelty and she lay in bed, crying her eyes out. Her family thought she was behaving very strangely but, in her

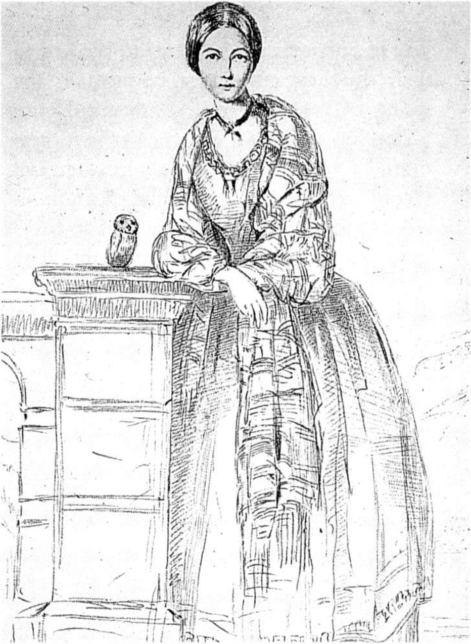

The young Florence

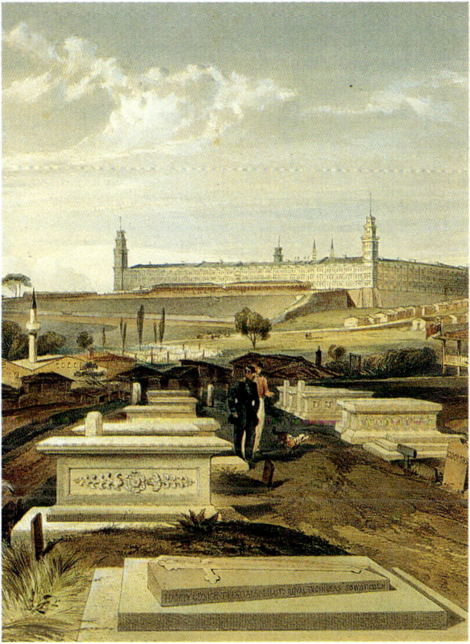

The hospital and cemetery at Scutari

to take an active part in the healing of the local villagers. But, with this aid, she came to realise the importance of professional training. She knew nothing and this came as a shock. It had always been universally assumed that the only qualification needed for nursing was to be female. Ignorance was total and its consequences fatal. She realised that she must receive technical training if she was to be of any real use and she conceived a plan to achieve this end.

She would persuade her parents to allow her to go for three months to Salisbury Infirmary to learn nursing : it was a well-known hospital and the head physician, Dr Fowler, was an old friend of the family with advanced views. In December 1845 the Fowlers came to stay and Florence seized her chance to propose her plan. Her parents were utterly horrified. W.E.N. went to London in a state of extreme disgust. Fanny could only think she must have conceived some attachment to a "low vulgar surgeon" and said as much. The Fowlers were acutely embarrassed by the whole scene and departed swiftly with Florence left defeated.

The Nightingales' reaction was not wholly surprising. In 1845 hospitals were places in which sick people became sicker. Beds were less than two feet apart and, as Florence was later to note, nurses never deigned to wash the patients who, thus, remained constantly filthy. New arrivals were put into the same sheets as the previous, generally deceased, occupants of their respective beds. It was virtually unknown for a respectable woman to become a hospital nurse – no decent woman could have borne such horror and degradation. The nurses slept in wooden cages on the landing places outside the doors of the wards, and it was impossible for any woman of character to sleep in such indecent surroundings. But Florence, at this stage, knew only that she had been humiliated and was now snubbed and lonely. She spent her nights praying to God and her days solemnly performing her filial duties. In her bedroom she developed a secret life of her own and began studying medical textbooks and sending away privately for medical reports and pamphlets. One of these was the Year Book of the Institution of Deaconesses at Kaiserswerth. She knew immediately that this was what she had been seeking. At the Institute she would be able to train as a nurse and none of the objections raised against English hospitals would apply. The religious atmosphere, the character of the deaconesses who formed the staff and the ascetic and disciplined lifestyle would place the home above suspicion. She hid the yearbook but retained the idea.

In Autumn 1847 the pressure was too much and she broke down completely. A new friend, Selina Bracebridge, and her ailing husband, Charles, took Florence to recuperate in Rome where she remained alone in the Sistine Chapel for a whole day and had the happiest New Year of her life. And then, in the winter of 1847, through the Bracebridges, she met the man who was to change her life – Sidney Herbert. He was good-looking, successful and unable to do wrong but he found the burden of his glittering career to be too much for him. He wanted something more from life and he and his wife, Liz, became devout Christians who consecrated their lives to philanthropic works. They built a church in their home town of Wilton and they devoted their lives to improving the condition of the poor. They had come to Rome to decide whether to become Roman Catholics. Florence herself began to go to mass every day and, after only a few months, she received what she believed to be a direct call from God to surrender her will to his completely. By May 1848, buoyed up by this experience, Florence returned to England but the Bracebriges took her abroad again, almost immediately, this time to Egypt. Florence was plagued with guilt. She considered that God was punishing her for being sinfully trivial and that this was why she was prevented from becoming a nurse. She writes in her diary:

May 12. Today I am 30 – the age Christ began his mission. Now no more childish things. No more love. No more marriage. Now Lord let me think only of Thy Will, what Thou willest me to do. Oh Lord Thy Will, Thy Will.

The Bracebridges were sensitive to Florence's delicate mental state and they realised that she would collapse unless they assisted her in her scheme. They brought her back from Egypt via Germany and, at last, left her at her long cherished Kaiserswerth in order for her to spend a fortnight examining the hospital and its facilities. She had entered a whole new world of medical care. The hospital did not smell. The apothecary was a woman. There were no resident male doctors and male patients were attended by male nurses. The whole experience was a

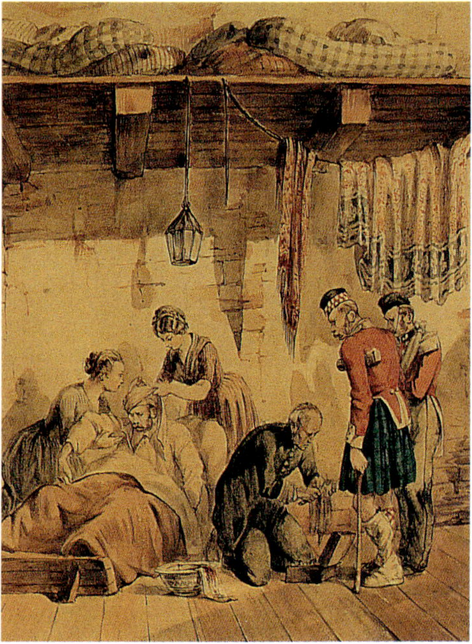

Nurses attend to new patients

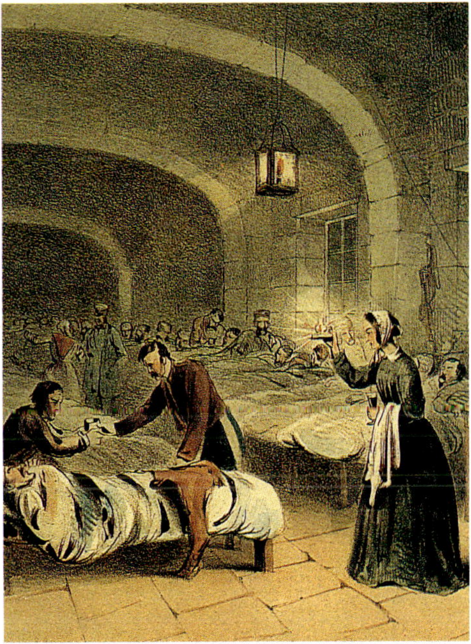

Florence Nightingale on her rounds

revelation to Florence and she wrote a pamphlet about her stay which Mr Bracebridge had printed and distributed anonymously. Florence was ecstatic but her happiness was temporary. She was soon to be returned home to a furiously angry mother and to a house in which the word 'Kaiserswerth' was never again to be mentioned. Henceforth, the struggle would be bitterer than ever.

Florence could bear no more and took her fate into her own hands. She declared that she would go whether her family liked it or not, and she made her own plans to go back to Kaiserswerth. Fanny could do nothing – her whole family was becoming ill over the affair – but insisted that the enterprise was shameful and forbade Florence to tell a soul about it. Parthe dashed herself into a frenzy over the affair and threw Florence's bracelets into her face. The scene was so violent that Florence fainted but she, nevertheless, got what she wanted. The following evening she reached Kaiserswerth.

Founded by a pastor in 1833, the hospital possessed, in 1851, one hundred beds, an infant school, an orphan asylum and a training school. Life was spartan and work was hard. Florence slept in the asylum and every minute of her day was accompanied by prayer. The Herberts came to visit and the founder of the institution himself told them that "no person had ever passed so distinguished an examination, or shown herself so thoroughly mistress of all she had to learn as Miss Nightingale". For the first time in her life, Florence was completely happy. On August 31, 1851, she wrote a long, humble letter to her family begging them to trust her and to help her. She wanted their blessing. Neither Fanny nor Parthe responded and Florence determined never to appeal to either of them again. Nonetheless, she had to come home.

In July 1852, ten months after her return, Florence was still confined to her home, her family bitterer than ever about her shameful behaviour. Fanny clung desperately to the hope that Florence would begin to behave like a normal young lady and get married, shutting her eyes to the fact that her daughter was thirty-two and had turned down all comers. Parthe verbally attacked Florence almost every day and worked herself up into hysterical frenzies. She declared that she was dying from mental agony and, a short while later, had a mental collapse, technically termed 'chronic delirium'. Taken to see a specialist, the Nightingales were told that Parthe's only chance of survival was to learn to survive away from her sister's overwhelming presence. In this totally unexpected way, Florence's fate was decided. In February she was sent away to Paris where she intended to enter a nunnery-hospital and undergo nursing training. She would wear a nun's habit and she would serve the sick. She was delighted with the prospect and spent a month in preparation, visiting hospitals and examining patients. Having already studied so diligently, Florence was already an expert. The day of her entry as a postulant approached when fate struck again and her grandmother died. Once again she was thwarted in her ambitions and forced to return to England.

Back in England, in April 1853, things began to look up. Liz Herbert wrote that she had heard that *The Institution for the Care of Sick Gentlewomen in Distressed Circumstances* was to be reorganised and its governing body, chaired by Lady Canning, was looking for a Superintendent to do the job. Liz suggested Florence as a candidate and, on being interviewed, she utterly charmed Lady Canning immediately and got the job. Parthe wept and raged; Fanny collapsed; W.E.N. retreated to his club, the Athenaeum, a broken man. On August 12, 1853 she went into residence in the new premises – Number 1, Harley Street.

Her ideas for immediate implementation were not merely highly demanding, they were revolutionary. She thought up a scheme for improved efficiency by having hot water pumped up to every floor. She organised a dumb waiter to bring the patients' food to their bedsides before it got cold. She wanted a bell for every bed, rigged to a system which would enable the nurses to know immediately which patient had rung. The committee was dazzled. They had never seen anything quite like it. All of the patients adored her and wrote extravagant letters of appreciation. She listened to their tales of loneliness, she sent the poorer women on day-trips to the seaside at her own expense and she wrote to relatives when the patients were too ill to do this for themselves. By January 1854 she was so well known that, when cholera broke out in London, Florence was asked to go immediately to the Middlesex Hospital in order to train the urgently required new nurses. She had reached a point of no return and was a celebrity when, in March 1854, England and France declared war on Russia. In September the Allies landed in the Crimea. War had begun.

# CRIMEA

Sidney Herbert was, by this time, the Secretary of State for War and he was, therefore, also responsible for the treatment of the sick and the wounded. Facilities in this area were criminally inadequate and, in the tremendous negative publicity that ensued, Sidney Herbert was held to be blameworthy. On October 15th he put into action his only remaining plan – he wrote to his old, and now famous friend, Florence Nightingale, and asked her to go to Scutari, in Turkey, and command a party of nurses. The expedition would have Government sanction and Government backing but, and this was critical to the enterprise, she was not being asked as an angel of mercy but as an efficient administrator of people. If her team acquitted themselves with flying colours then nurses would never be despised again. A lot of Florence's greatest ambitions were at stake.

Forty nurses were to be chosen and Florence was appointed "Superintendent of the Female Nursing Establishment of the English General Hospitals in Turkey". Her authority would extend to distribution of nurses, hours of attendance, allotment to duties and selection of staff. The appointment caused a sensation. No woman had ever before held such a distinguished position. At last Fanny and Parthe gushed with enthusiasm. They raised no objection to her chosen path now that she was famous and highly lauded. The headquarters for recruitment would be the Herberts' London home in Belgrave Square and the standard of volunteers was pitiful. Florence did not kid herself about the ordinary woman's motivation for going : "One alone expressed a wish to go from a good motive." she said, "Money was the only inducement".

Florence drew up a list of rules. Misconduct would be punishable with immediate dismissal. No young women were acceptable. Each nurse was to be provided with a uniform but was to bring her own underclothing, four cotton night-caps, one cotton umbrella and a carpet-bag. No coloured ribbons or flowers were allowed. Under

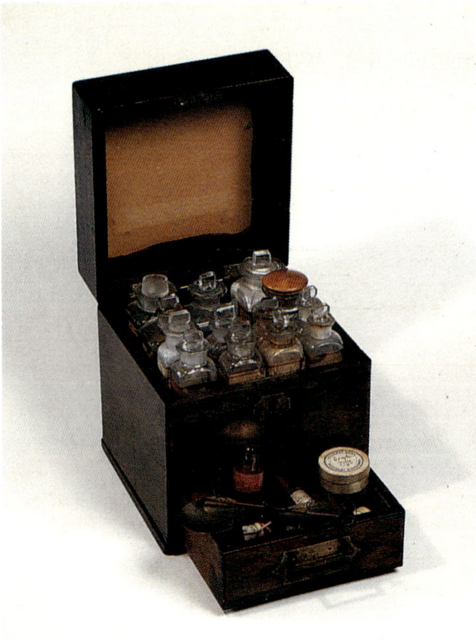

Florence Nightingale's medicine chest

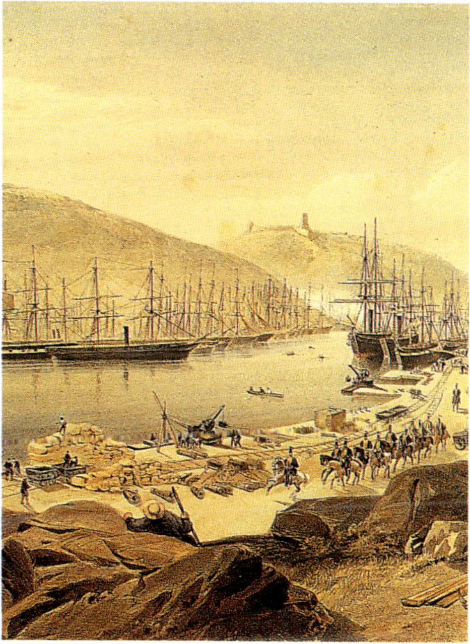

The harbour at Balaclava

no circumstances were the nurses permitted to to go out unaccompanied at night. No nurse was to leave the hospital without permission. Strong liquor was permitted in only moderate quantities. The demands were tough and only fourteen professional nurses could be found to fit the criteria; the remaining twenty-four were all members of religious institutions.

On October 21, 1854, the party left London Bridge to travel to Paris via Boulogne where they were greeted with mass applause at Boulogne. The landlord refused to accept any money and Florence waited on the nurses herself. At Paris the party was cheered all the way to their hotel. The women were stars. They travelled down to Marseilles and then sailed in the *Vectis* for Constantinople. On November 3rd they rushed up the Bosphorus and anchored. Lord Stratford, the British Ambassador at Constantinople, sent Lord Napier, the Secretary, to greet the party. He found Florence stretched out on a sofa, riddled with sea-sickness from the journey, but, immediately and just like everyone else she encountered at this time, he was utterly captivated by her presence and force of personality.

The nurses were to go to the cavernous Barrack Hospital at once. Wending their muddy way up the detritus filled alleys towards the hospital, the nurses shrank back in horror. The voyage was horrific but the destination was even worse. There were four miles of beds; every corner of every room was in a state of utter disrepair; the courtyard in the centre of the barracks was filled with rubbish and rotting corpses;

one whole side of the building had been gutted by fire. The basement of the building was inhabited by 200 disease-ridden women who were, either as wives, mothers or prostitutes, attached to the army in some ill-defined and undisciplined way. This wasn't a hospital; it was hell and, in this hell, 1,400 of the 2,400 patients were reported incapacitated by alcohol.

The British troops who fell sick at Sebastopol and were brought to Scutari, died there as a result of malnourishment, filth and overcrowding. Winter was approaching and each week the number of sick rose. The entire British Army's health was run by one man with no budget and a staff of four. His job was under-paid and despised but, even run by the most worthy of men, it would have been considered impertinent for a mere officer to suggest changes. The position was stagnant and men were, consequently, dying. Systems of supply were negligible; there were shortages of the greatest magnitude and officers were trained not to make any trouble. Each and every requisition involved obtaining four signatures. It was impossible to achieve a thing.

But none of this was assisted by the fact that the ordinary soldier was considered, at this period, totally unworthy of respect. The Duke of Wellington, whose victories were due largely to these despised men, described his army as "the scum of the earth enlisted for drink". Officers hardly considered their staff as human at all and Florence was officially informed not to spoil or pamper them. All of the doctors considered Florence's appointment to be a folly of the highest

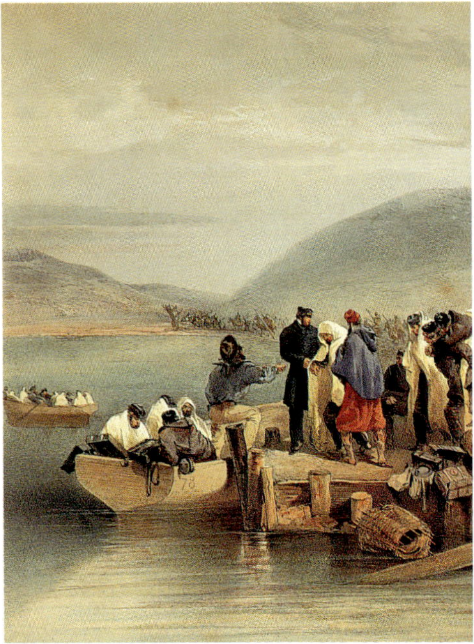


Embarkation of the wounded at Balaclava

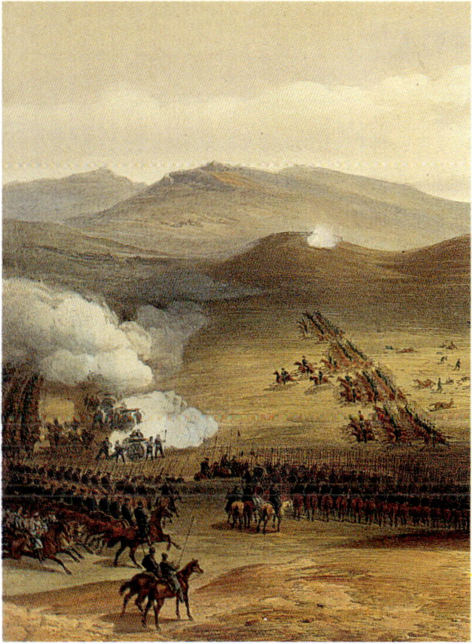

*The Charge of the Light Cavalry Brigade*

order. A group of delicate young plants led by a leading society lady could not possibly be anything except an added burden to them. But they had no choice. On November 5th the party was welcomed into the hospital with hypocritical goodwill whilst the doctors considered Florence Nightingale to be, at best, burdensome and, at worst, a government spy. They did their best to make the women as physically unwelcome as possible. All forty were to live in six rooms, each one more filthy and unhygenic than the next. There was no furniture and little food. One of the rooms contained the rotting corpse of a Russian general but they were given no equipment with which to clean it away. And there were no beds. Florence, to her horror, discovered that this was the least of her problems – there were also no operating tables and no medical supplies and there was very little water or wax. At least, she joked, they wouldn't have to stare at the rats.

As the days wore on, the doctors continued to ignore Florence and refuse her supplies. Offers of help from her nurses were rejected out of hand and Florence, though she wished things were otherwise, realised that she would never achieve anything unless she received the co-operation of the doctors who hated her. She had to convince them that she didn't wish to undermine their authority and that they would always retain control of their own hospital. She determined that that no nurse would be allowed onto the wards until she had personal knowledge of their competence and she began to make small steps towards establishing her position.

The day after Florence arrived she transformed one room in her nurses' quarters into an extra kitchen. Previously there had been a mere thirteen saucepans in the entire building and only one kitchen with no cutlery. She began to cook arrowroot, wine and beef broth which she had brought with her and this small detail made an immediate improvement to the diets of those lucky few who were fed from her kitchen rather than the main one. But this also caused problems since the others naturally became very resentful.

On November 9th the battle situation worsened so considerably that differences between the parties were temporarily forgotten. The annihilation of the British Army had begun. Surviving soldiers suffered from scurvy, starvation and exposure to the Crimean winter. The only road to the British base in the area, Balaclava, had been taken over by the Russians on October 25th. The town had become a cesspool. The great majority of soldiers had cholera and piles of arms and legs, amputated after the battle of Balaclava, had been chucked into the shallow harbour of the town where they remained putrid and permanently visible. The whole town reeked of disease and sick men began pouring into the hospital in overwhelming numbers. The majority of the men were suffering from diarrhoea and they had only twenty chamber pots between them. Those wounded who were not sick with fever all became so and, to make matters yet worse, on November 14th the worst hurricane ever to be seen in the area, struck the whole region.

And, like much of her life pattern, it was this unexpected calamity which transformed Florence's fortunes. The staff of the hospital suddenly realised to whom they could turn for help – Florence Nightingale. She had over £30,000 at her disposal and no-one else had a penny. In the hour of greatest need it was money which gave Florence the power base she had been seeking for weeks. The doctors had no choice – if any men were to survive they would have to kow-tow to the infuriatingly well-off Florence. Immediately, she commandeered the staff. She took over the purveyor's records and she established which articles were most urgently needed. She made lists of required objects and she sent men into Constantinople to buy them. Her very first order was scrubbing-brushes for the floors. She insisted that each of the tub-baths in the wards was emptied, for the first time ever, and then washed out. She rented a house outside the barracks and commissioned the soldiers' wives to do the washing – the first time this had ever happened. She paid for boilers to be installed and then purchased 6,000 shirts, 2,000 socks and 500 pairs of underpants. She bought in essential winter clothing for entire regiments – all of which had hitherto been considered impossible.

At the beginning of December 500 more sick and wounded were brought in to the hospital. There was simply no more room. Florence, out of her own personal funds, engaged 200 workmen and had the whole burnt wing of the hospital restored, refurbished and reequipped. "We felt we were in heaven", said one of the soldiers, who had never seen anything like it. The news of the

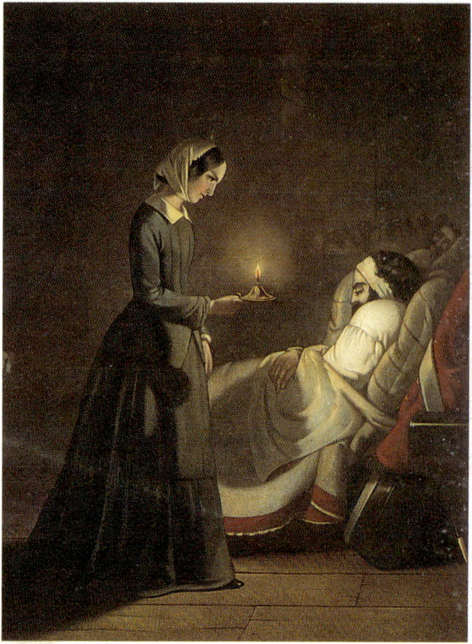

'The lady with the lamp'

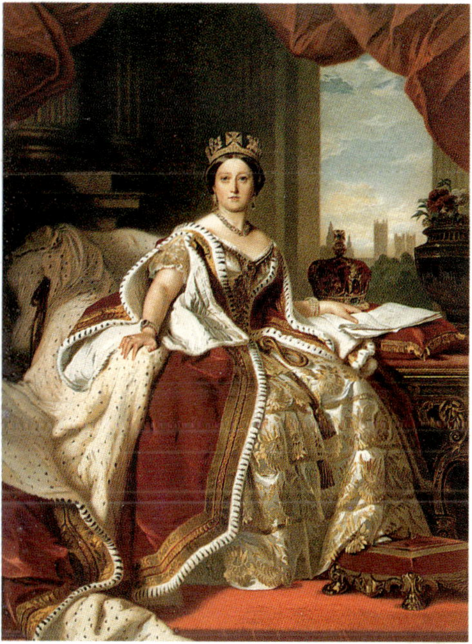

Queen Victoria

work caused a sensation, particularly when it was discovered by local colonels that the money she spent had been refunded to her by the government but, and most importantly, despite her tremendous success, Florence never forgot the fact that the original aim of the voyage was to prove the value of women as nurses. They did not however always assist her in this aim.

One of the nuns wrote a letter home describing the fearful state of the wards and this was passed on to *The Times* by her family which published it as part of their vigorous campaign to discredit the government. Florence was horrified, both by the disloyalty of the nurse and by the negative impression the letter would create on the doctors whom she had been trying so hard to impress. There was an official enquiry and the nun was proved to be lying and asked to resign but her attitude was commonplace and she had more friends amongst the nurses than Florence herself. It was commonly recognised that many of them actively disliked Miss Nightingale for her perceived callousness and single-minded ambition.

Between December 17 and January 3, 4,000 more patients were brought to the hospital. One of the officers wrote to Sidney Herbert at this time that "Flo has been working herself to death, never sits down to breakfast or dinner without interruption: often never dines . . . the attempt to do more will kill her . . . today 200 sick landed looking worse than any others yet." And yet one of the nurses reported that as far as looks and power went, she had never seen Florence looking better. Her position was strengthened by a letter sent by Queen Victoria to Sidney Herbert : "Would you tell Mrs Herbert that I beg she would let me see frequently the accounts she receives from Miss Nightingale . . . Let Mrs Herbert also know that I wish Miss Nightingale and the ladies would tell these poor noble wounded and sick men that no-one takes a warmer interest or feels more for their sufferings or admires their courage and heroism more than their Queen." The soldiers were thrilled. The message was read out loud to them in the wards and the Queen sent them all Christmas gifts. Florence, now in an unshakeable position of strength, wrote directly to the Queen asking her, amongst other things, to regulate pay for the sick soldiers and to reorganise the local cemeteries. The Queen was delighted to assist her new heroine and acted immediately upon both requests. All those men who had previously opposed Florence now realised what a truly powerful position she held.

On January 2nd, 1,200 more men arrived at once. By spring 1855 she was exhausted. She lived in impossible conditions and tended the sick for twenty-four hours at a stretch. It was her golden rule never to let a man die alone. Most of the time she had to fulfil this aim herself, witnessing the deaths of over 2,000 men personally and, for each man, she held the same extraordinary, charismatic hypnotism.

"What a comfort it was to see her pass even", wrote one soldier, "We lay there by hundreds; but we could kiss her shadow as it fell and lay our heads on the pillow again content". But some of the joy had gone out of her work with the official end to the crisis. Her daily life now consisted of tedious administration; official intrigue and petty jealousy, though the mortality rate dropped consistently. Sanitation was improved beyond recognition; there were plenty of supplies and diet had been revolutionised by the appearance of Alexis Soyer, a world-famous chef, who had arrived in March 1855, to do his bit for Britain and Florence. Now that the Barrack Hospital was under control, Florence determined to go to the Crimean frontline itself. She had, however, been appointed Superintendent only in Turkey. She discovered much to her bitter chagrin, that she had no jurisdiction over the battle zone. Florence, never one to be put off by fixed regulations, decided to go anyway and, on May 5th, along with Soyer, the chef, and other specially selected members of her entourage, she arrived in Balaclava. The news spread like wildfire and the soldiers rushed from their tents to greet their goddess of mercy. She ignored the hostility of the local authorities and began an inspection. Florence was determined to transform Balaclava as she had Scutari but, before she could put this new plan into action, she collapsed with Crimean fever. The whole army was in uproar at the news. Men wept on hearing the news – for them she was their sole representative of hope.

Queen Victoria wrote expressing her deep concern. Florence's health was a national disaster. Everyone begged her to come home but, on improving a little, she decided merely to return to Scutari. However, whilst she was being nursed to health,

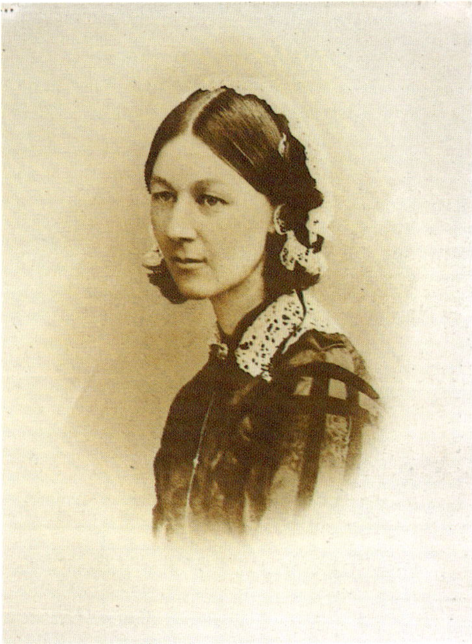

Florence Nightingale pictured on her visiting card

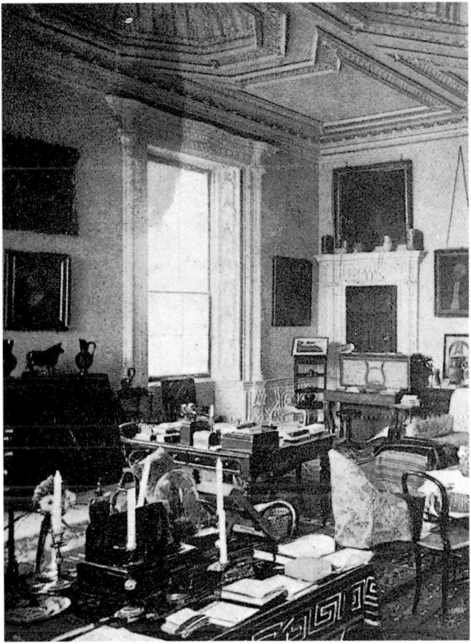

Florence's room at her sister's house, Claydon

she temporarily lost control over her nurses, who proceeded to get drunk, pregnant or simply to die. Some ran home and claimed to have been ill-treated. Pressure began to mount on Florence. On September 8th Sebastopol fell and the end of the war was merely a matter of time but reports started to appear in the British press to the effect that the British army was incapable of looking after itself and that it had needed Florence Nightingale, a mere woman, to rescue it single-handed. The harm done was tremendous since the army doctors thought that Florence had started the campaign herself. To top it all, she was taken ill again and so, by November, she found herself in the astonishing position of being a national heroine at home but loathed and detested in the Crimea.

In Britain she was already a legend. Songs were written about her; biographies sold like hotcakes; ceramics were moulded bearing her portrait. The Nightingale Fund was formed and Queen Victoria had a brooch engraved specially for Florence who was, herself, not particularly moved by all this praise. It became clear to her, with the end of the war approaching, that she must improve the lot of the soldier in peace as well as in war and she became mystically devoted to this cause. She started a literacy club for the soldiers in the hospital and she wrote to the Queen about the alcohol problem. She had the local drink shops closed down and started, instead, a coffee house from private funds. Four schools were opened and singing classes formed. By January 1856 the image of the British soldier as a drunken lout had vanished but all this good work came at a

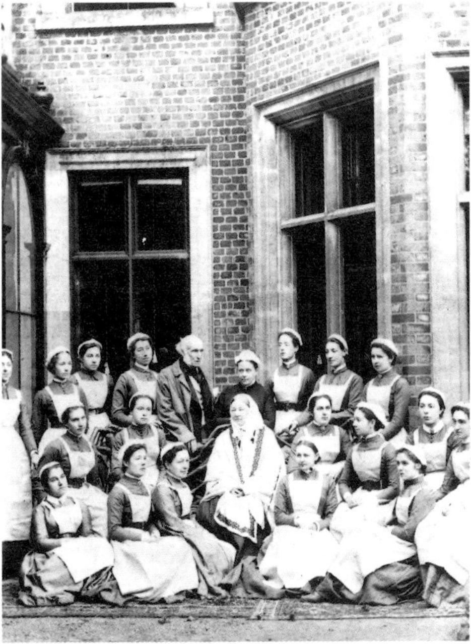

Florence and her nurses at Claydon

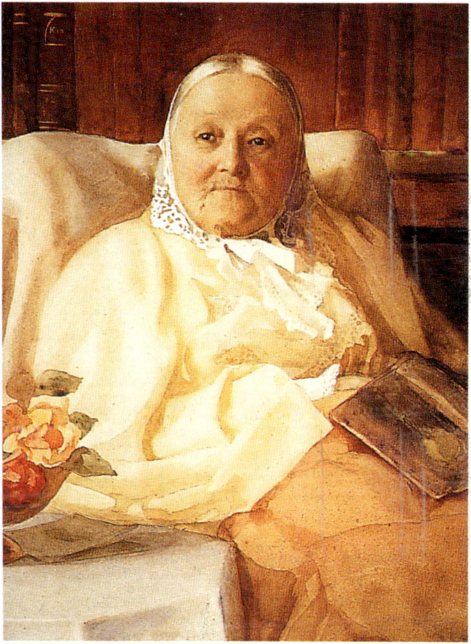

Florence Nightingale in 1909

Paris with her old friend, Clarkey, and then she continued on to England, alone. She took the train north and walked, unannounced, from the station to Lea Hurst. Parthe, Fanny and W.E.N. were in the drawing-room chatting quietly when she walked in without any fuss. Whilst she had single-handedly brought about a social revolution, she had ended the Crimean War with a sense of her own personal failure.

# LATER YEARS

After Crimea Florence never again made a public appearance or attended a function. Her postbag was enormous but it was Parthe who opened her mail and replied. Early in September an old friend, Sir James Clark, wrote inviting her to stay in his Scottish retreat which was only a mile from Balmoral. Queen Victoria had requested to meet her in person. Florence knew what she must do. She would ask for a Royal Commission to be set up and to examine the sanitation and organisation of the Army Medical Department – now she would devote her time to reforming the lot of the average, peacetime soldier. The meeting with the Queen lasted for over two hours. It was a grand success.

"She put before us," wrote the Prince, "all the defects of our present military hospital system and the reforms that are needed. We are much pleased with her; she is extremely modest." She was asked back again and again. The relevant people were informed, letters were written, communications sent and then, of course, nothing actually happened. The official announcement of the issue of the Royal Warrant to set up the Commission never transpired. By March 1st 1857 Florence was in despair. The War Office wrote her memorandum after memorandum but she had no faith in their intentions. She thought that they meant to carry on their placating communications forever. She held back the publicity card but she realised that she might be forced to use it. She had one last trick up her sleeve and wrote to the government threatening to expose all of the inefficiency she had observed in Crimea unless she got her way immediately. Where royal influence had failed, blackmail worked. Every request she made was granted. On May 5th 1857 the Royal Warrant was issued and the following week the Commission began to sit – and it was now composed of people she had personally chosen.

She was the central figure in the inquiry. The men in the Commission called her the Commander-in-Chief. She collected all the information and collated it and then wrote down her conclusions. Before each witness appeared she would prepare a questionnaire with the relevant facts to be elicited. She personally coached Sidney Herbert, the Chairman, before each interview and, at his request, saw every one of the witnesses herself prior to the Commission. By July it was time for the most important witness of all – Florence herself. Sidney Herbert did not wish her to raise the Crimea issue, since he did not want unnecessary controversy and so, for the general good of the Commission she restricted herself to written answers but she wrote as no-one had ever written before. The soldier was a human being for whom life had value, she stated, and, clearly, a decent quality of life would make for a better fighting man. Brutalised men do not make better fighters, she stated (and at the time this was revelatory) but worse.

By January 1858 Florence was exhausted but continued to work herself to the bone. Sir Harry Verney, a fifty-six year old pioneer in rural housing and an immensely handsome man, suddenly appeared in her life and fell madly in love with her. As ever, she refused his hand but he was not deterred by this rejection and decided to fall in love with her sister instead. He was already a widower with three children and so, at the age of thirty-nine, Parthe quietly and without fuss, became Lady Verney. Florence was delighted. At long last she would be left in peace. She moved into a private annex of the Burlington Hotel where everyone was convinced that she was so fragile she would shortly die. She made arrangements for her own funeral and wrote a will in which the estate she would eventually inherit from her parents would be converted into a model barracks.

She visited no-one but dozens of eminent people came to call : the Queen of Holland, the Crown Princess of Prussia and the Duke of Cambridge. But these were wearying times. Her old friend and chef, Alexis Soyer died whilst working with her on plans for a model army kitchen and Sidney Herbert became too unwell to do any work – which was a disaster since he was chairman of all four sub-committees on the Commission. At the end of Summer 1859, Florence herself collapsed with fainting, breathlessness and inability to eat. She stayed in bed continuously and even caused a family feud since, when the Verneys came to London, she claimed to be too sick to see them. The maids apparently reported to Parthe that Florence was relatively well. Everywhere she turned, Florence began to see disaster but she carried on with what she saw as the crucial issues and continued to publish pamphlets.

She expanded her ideas into a book called *Notes on Hospitals* which was very successful and went into a third edition. Following its success she was asked for advice on hospital construction and many of the designs of Victorian hospitals were specifically dictated by her and, in 1859, St Thomas's Hospital appealed to her directly for help. It was, at that time situated in Borough and a railway company wanted to buy the site for a station. No-one knew what to do about this thorny issue and Florence was called upon to decide. She had always taken an interest in the hospital since her chief nurse in the Crimea, Mrs Roberts, had been a sister there. Unlike anyone else involved in the project, Florence did specific research involving the newly founded science of statistics and she discovered that very few of the patients at the hospital were actually locals. Most came from poorer neighbourhoods South of the river and so she advised, and naturally her advice was followed, that the whole site be sold and a new hospital built at its present site in Lambeth. She decided to use a large sum from the Nightingale Fund to set up a nursing school at the hospital and she wrote the first textbook for the new school herself – *Notes on Nursing* was published in January 1860.

What would be plain common sense nowadays was revelatory stuff at the time. Florence attacked the ignorance of Victorian girls about their own bodies as shameful and, rather shockingly, she encouraged every woman to wash regularly. The book was quite expensive for the time but 15,000 copies were sold within a month and thousands of copies were distributed to schools and factories and it was translated into French, German and Italian.

In May 1860 the first applications were considered for the training school. Fifteen candidates were selected and the rules were explained to them before the opening of the school in July 1860. No pupil was to be admitted without a certificate of good character. Training was to last for a whole year – which was an extraordinary length of time. The nurses were to live in a 'home' – a revolutionary concept – and they were to wear a special brown uniform. Each probationer was given £10 for personal expenses and, at the end of the year, each satisfactory student was to be awarded a certificate with financial rewards dependent on how well each student had fared in her end of year report under the headings 'Moral Record' and 'Technical Record'.

Meanwhile, in June 1861 Sidney Herbert wrote to Florence to tell her that he could bear the pressure no longer and that he intended to resign. Florence was outraged and refused to believe that he was ill. She cut him off and refused to speak to him. He came to see her and she told him, mercilessly, that he was a failure both as a parliamentarian and as a man. He went away heartbroken and within a month he was dead. Florence was mortified. She refused ever to go back to her rooms in the Burlington Hotel and moved to Hampstead where she would see no-one. All of Sidney's work on her behalf began to be undone and she was convinced that her life's mission had ended. Her endlessly open door to the government had been closed and, for several weeks, she expected nothing more than to die but, by January 1862, she had begun to improve and she moved into the Verneys' London home in Mayfair.

As an advisor her position was unshakeable but her influence was never to be quite the same again. For the next four years every problem affecting the British army was referred to her for an opinion, though her advice was rarely actually taken. She had become the Elder Statesman on military and hospital affairs and yet she was convinced, by this stage, that everyone hated her except her cats. She felt that they were the only beings with whom she had any sympathy: "Dumb beasts observe you so much more than human beings and know so much better what you are thinking of", she wrote in 1862, now feeling utterly alone.

Florence found a new cause to keep her spirits up temporarily – professional training for midwives – which had been, up till now, something that women "just knew how to do". Although popular opinion, in general, was moving towards women being allowed to train as doctors, Florence was not interested. There were plenty of excellent doctors already, she claimed, but there were still very few competent nurses and midwives. In 1862 Dr Elizabeth Blackwell became the first woman to qualify as a doctor and, with this, a celebrity. Florence remained uninterested. "The women have made no improvement," she wrote, "they have only tried to be 'men' and they have succeeded only in being third rate men."

She set up a lengthy correspondence with the philosopher John Stuart Mill who laboured to convince her of the need for female enfranchisement. In July 1867 he asked her to become a member of the first committee of the London National Society for Women's Suffrage. She refused, not apparently because she was not interested but because she thought that there were much more pressing concerns to be dealt with than the right to vote. She could not believe that giving women the vote would do anything to improve their lot – this could only happen with a general and comprehensive improvement in national economic conditions. She was now forty-eight and considered herself old and then, in March

1868, the Tories lost the election and the Liberals, with Gladstone as their leader, came into power. Gladstone and Florence had always loathed each other. She was losing power on all sides and, for the first time in her life, she had no energy to fight on.

In the summer of 1869 she went to stay with her parents for the first time in years. She read novels (her favourite author was Jane Austen) and she chatted to her father. By 1872 she was spending eight months of the year at her family home. She wrote: "Never has God let me feel weariness of active life, but only anxiety to get on. Now in old age I never wish to be relieved from new work, but only to have it to do." Fanny was now blind and suffering from senile dementia. W.E.N. was seventy-nine and could not cope. Florence was desperately bored but felt she had to stay and help and in 1874 her father finally died. The house now belonged to an aunt and Fanny might be turned out of her own home. Parthe said she thought her mother should go and live in London and Florence felt utterly oppressed. "Not a day passes without the most acute anxiety and care. Oh the cruel waste of time of all real work . . . How happy it was in the Crimea on account of these things; that was living in spite of misery". Florence had reached the most awful period of her life. She felt totally shipwrecked but release was, eventually, to hand and in 1880 Fanny finally died at the age of ninety-two.

A change came over Florence. At last she could begin to look to the future again and, fortuitously, just as she felt she might once again start to hope, new opportunities arose.

She regained some influence in the War Office and in 1884, when the Gordon Relief Expedition was sent to Egypt, female nurses were officially sent out by the government and Florence was chosen to select the staff and organise the committee. Her health improved; she went to the opening of the new law courts and Queen Victoria spoke to her, saying that she was glad to see her looking so well.

In 1879 the British Nurses Association published a manifesto declaring their intention to formalise nurses' training under one general practice certificate. Florence violently disapproved : the object of this training would be pure technical knowhow and the important part of being a nurse was the attainment of moral standards which could not be gained by examination. The result